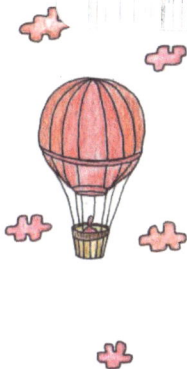

This book belongs to:

_____

_____

_____

First Published in Australia in 2021
Text and illustrations copyright
© Alice Pulvers, 2021

ISBN 978-0-6488917-5-8

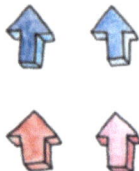

Feeling Blue?

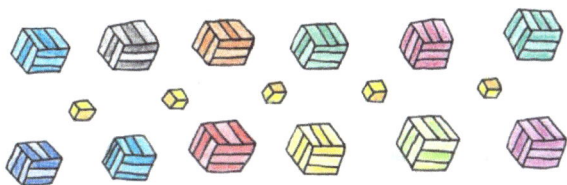

A book to help you
find colour in your day

by Alice Pulvers

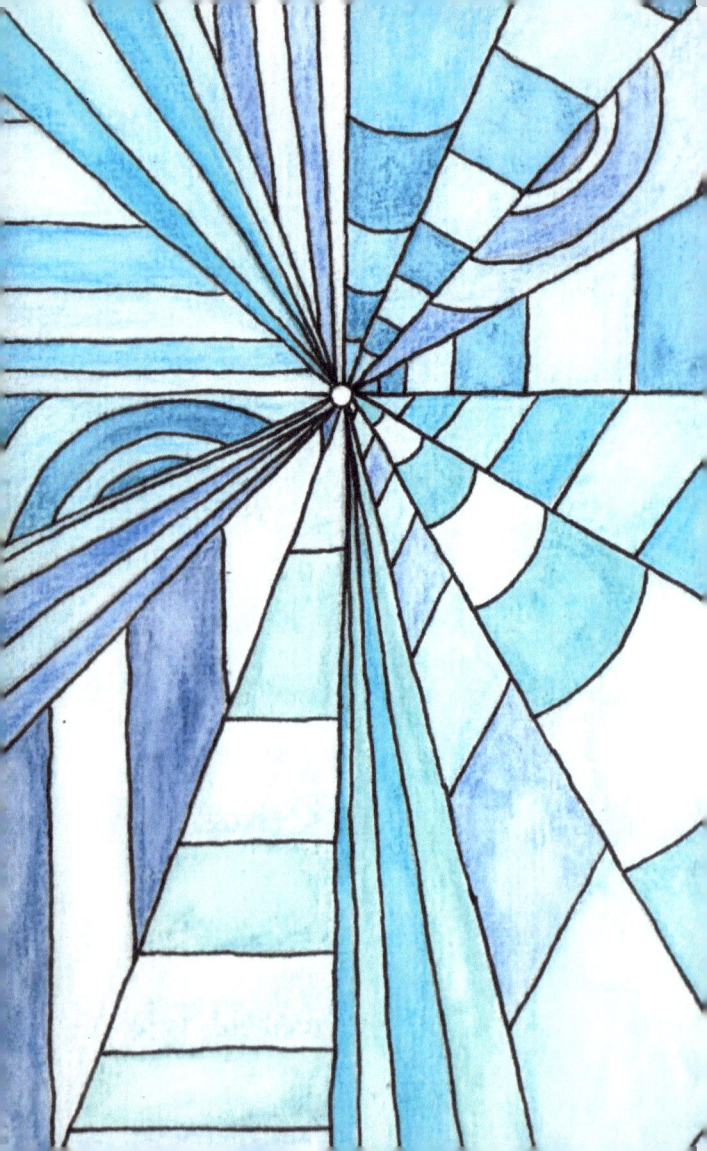

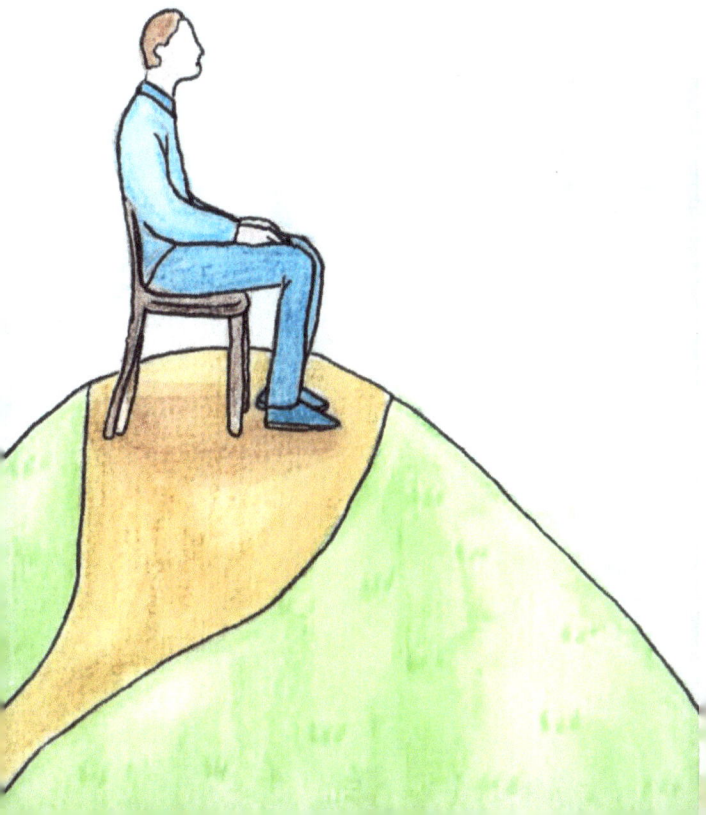

The sky is blue

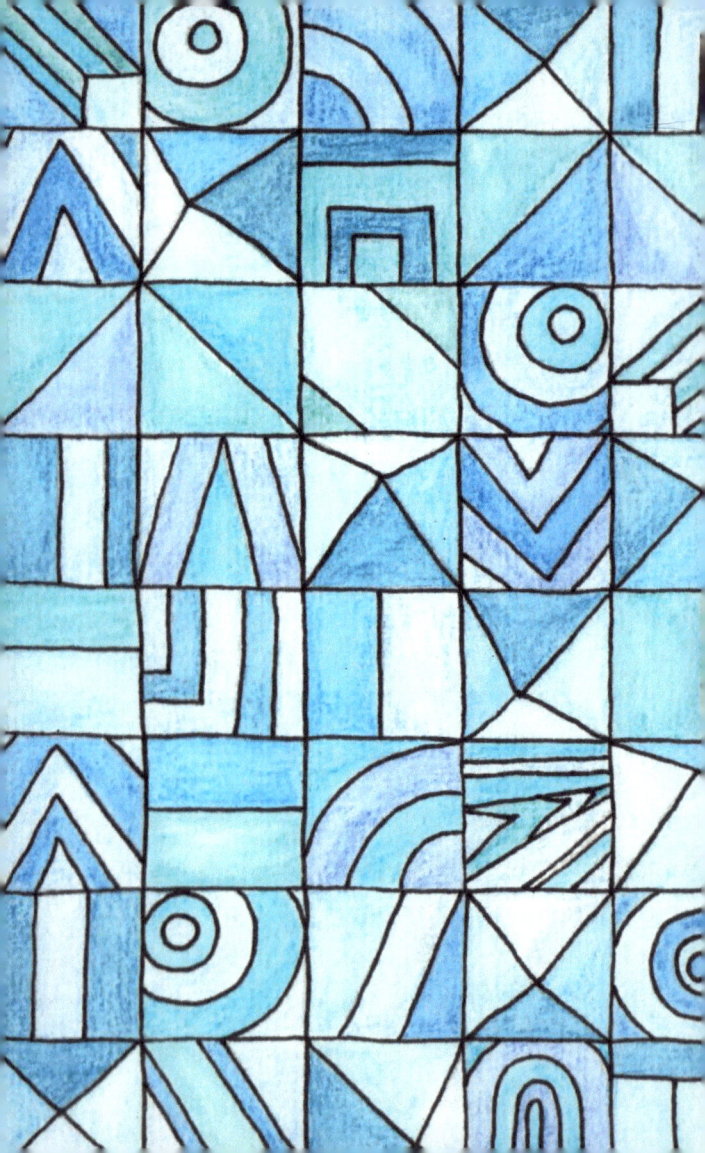

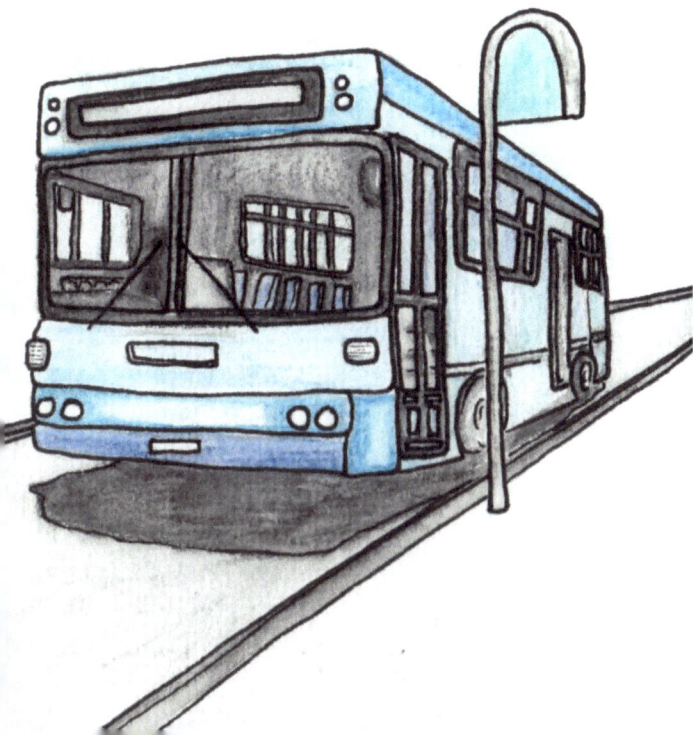

My bus is blue

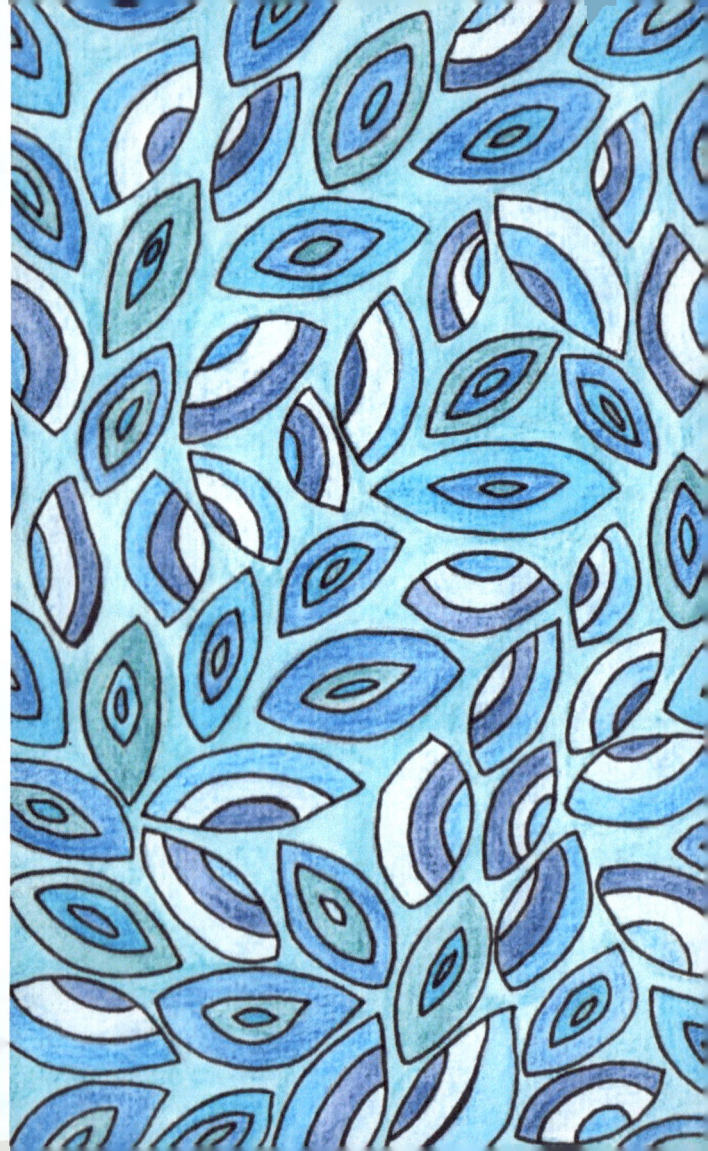

The bag on my
back is a darker
shade of blue

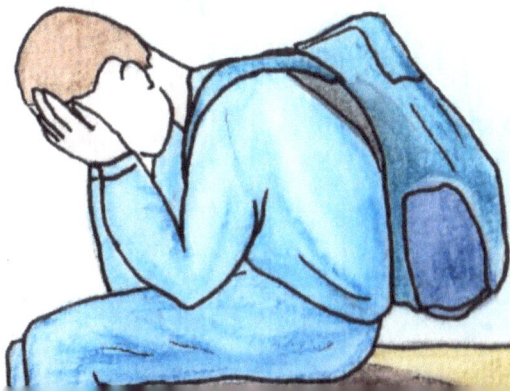

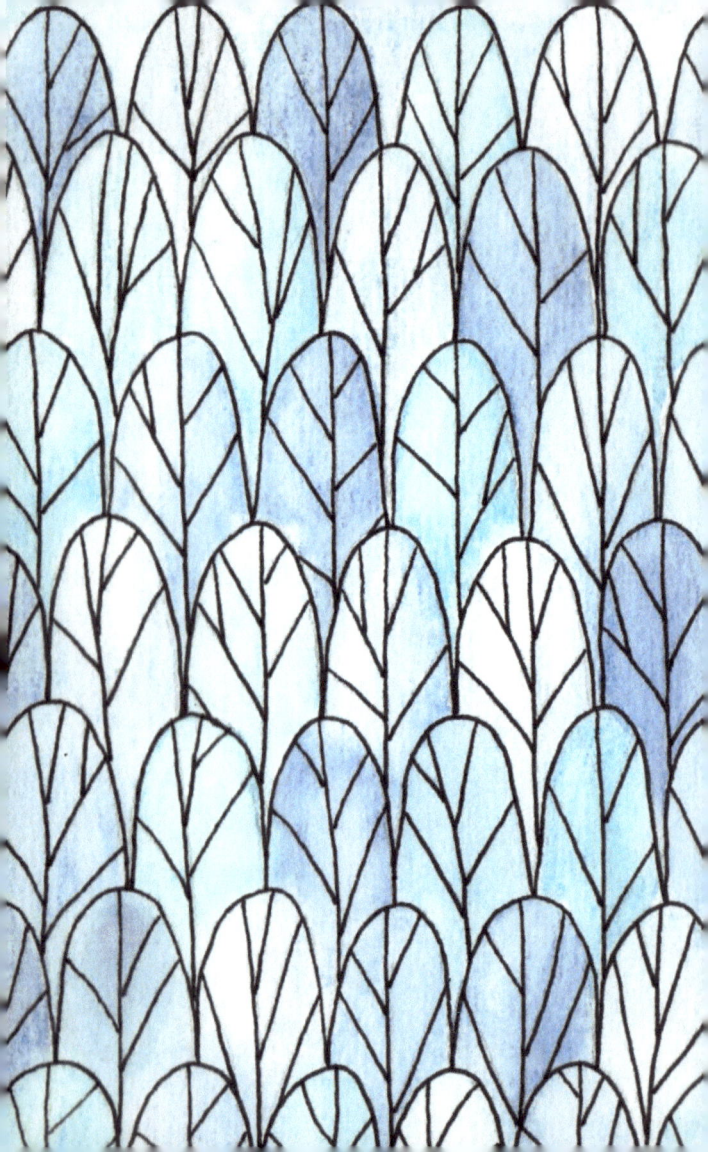

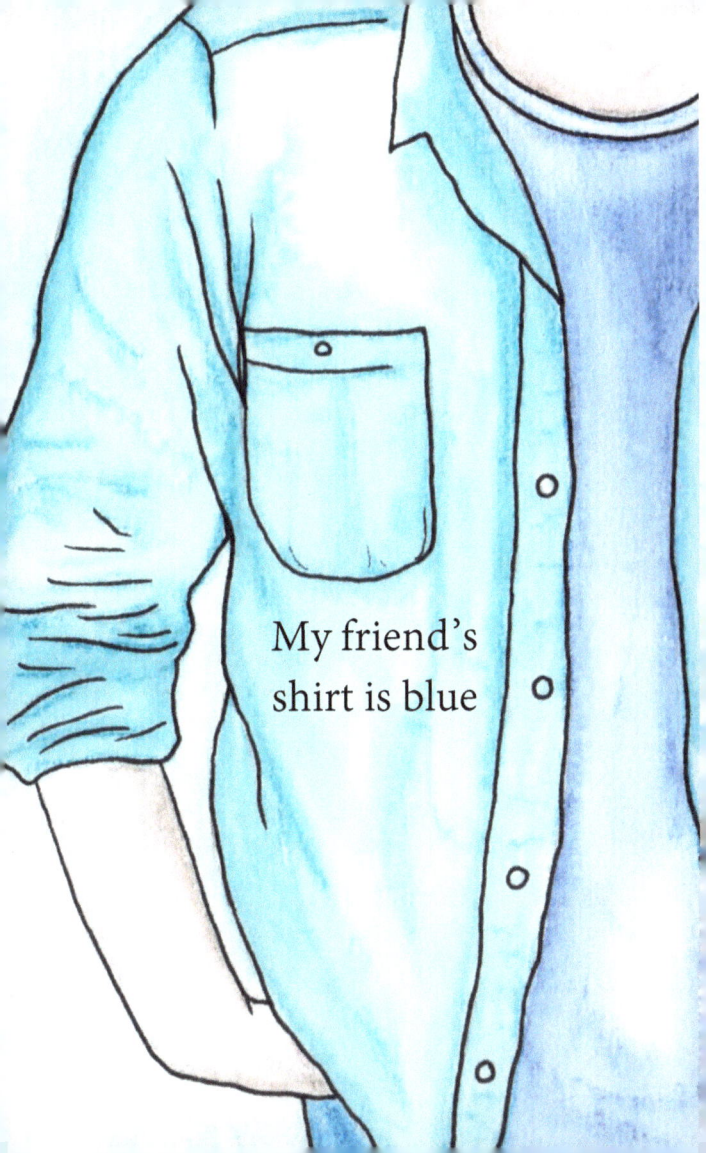

My friend's
shirt is blue

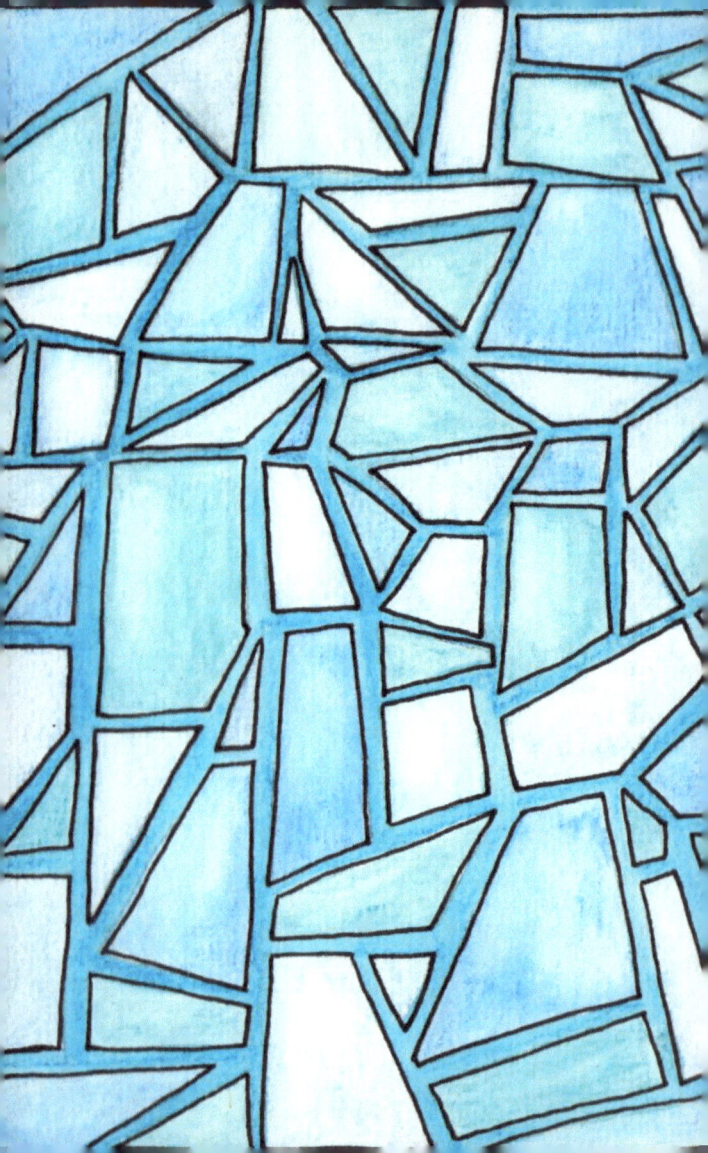

But why do I feel blue …

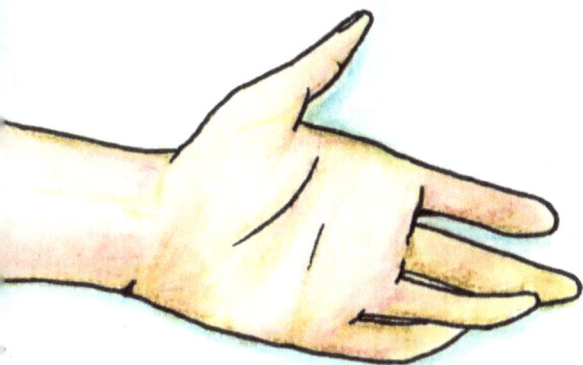

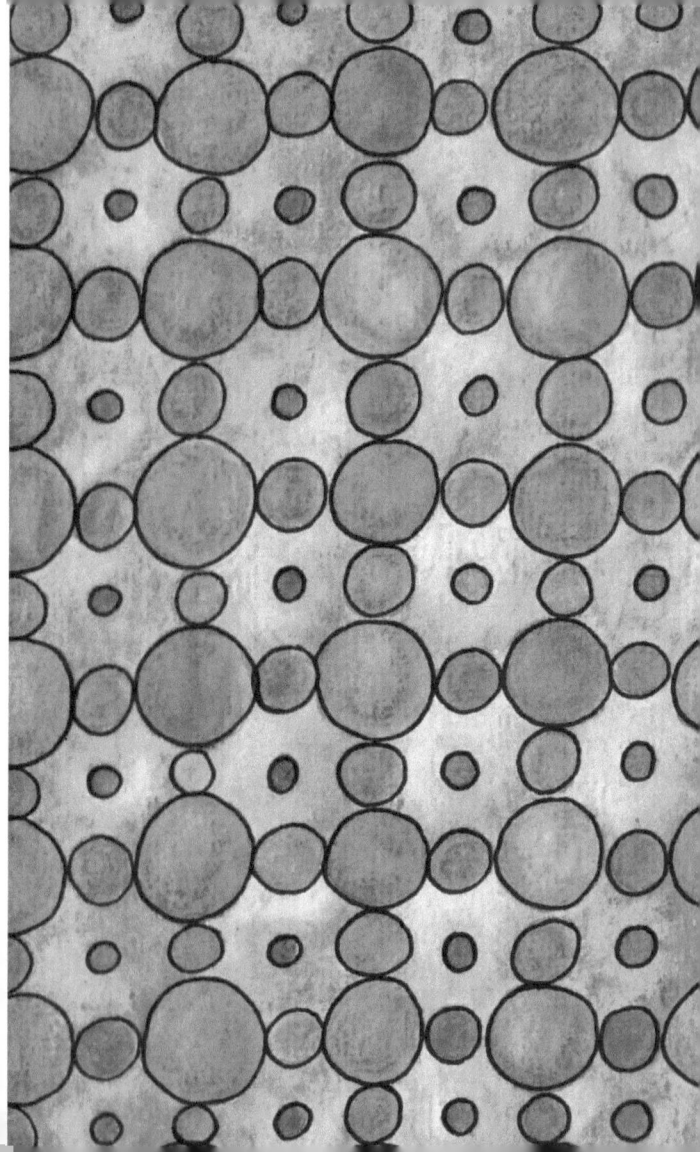

The afternoon sky is pink

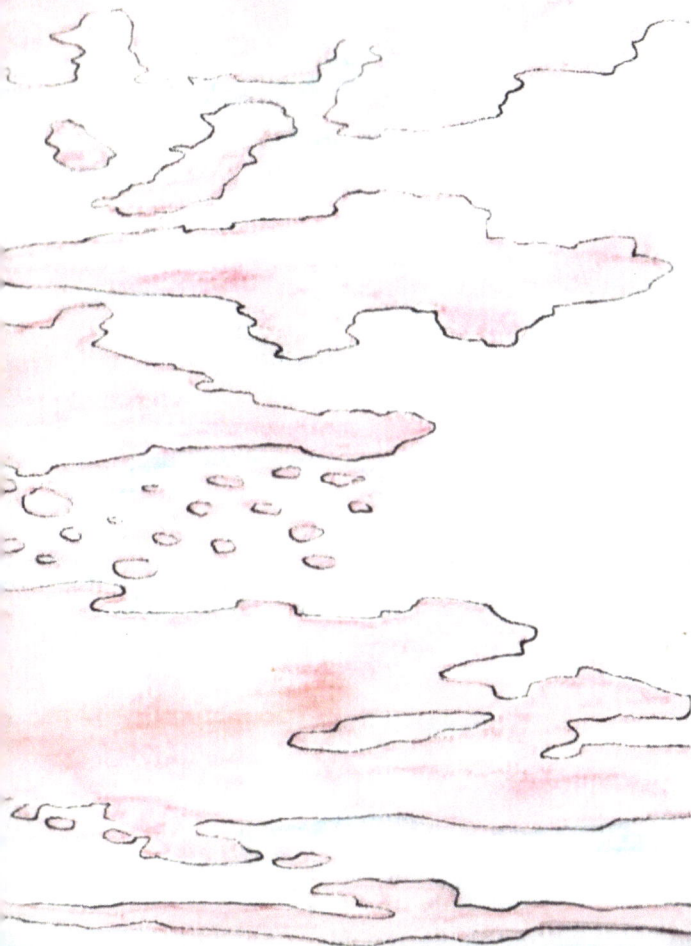

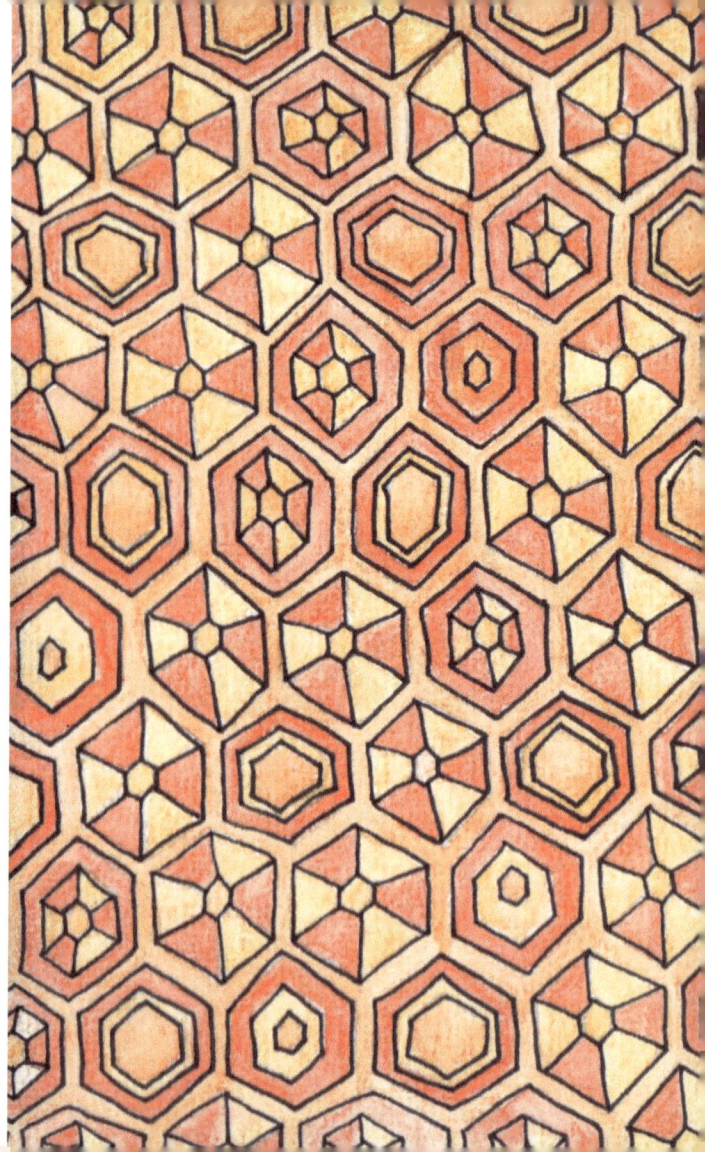

I see orange cats
through a window

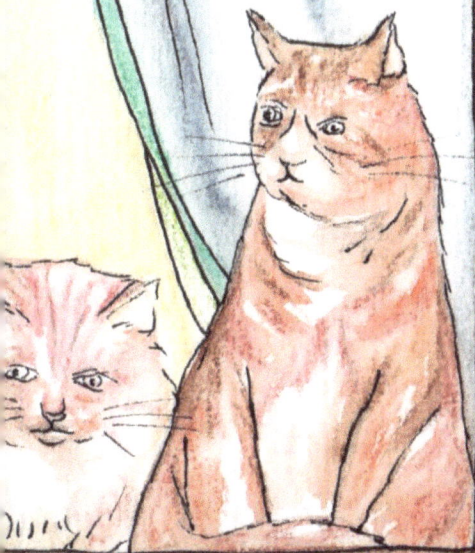

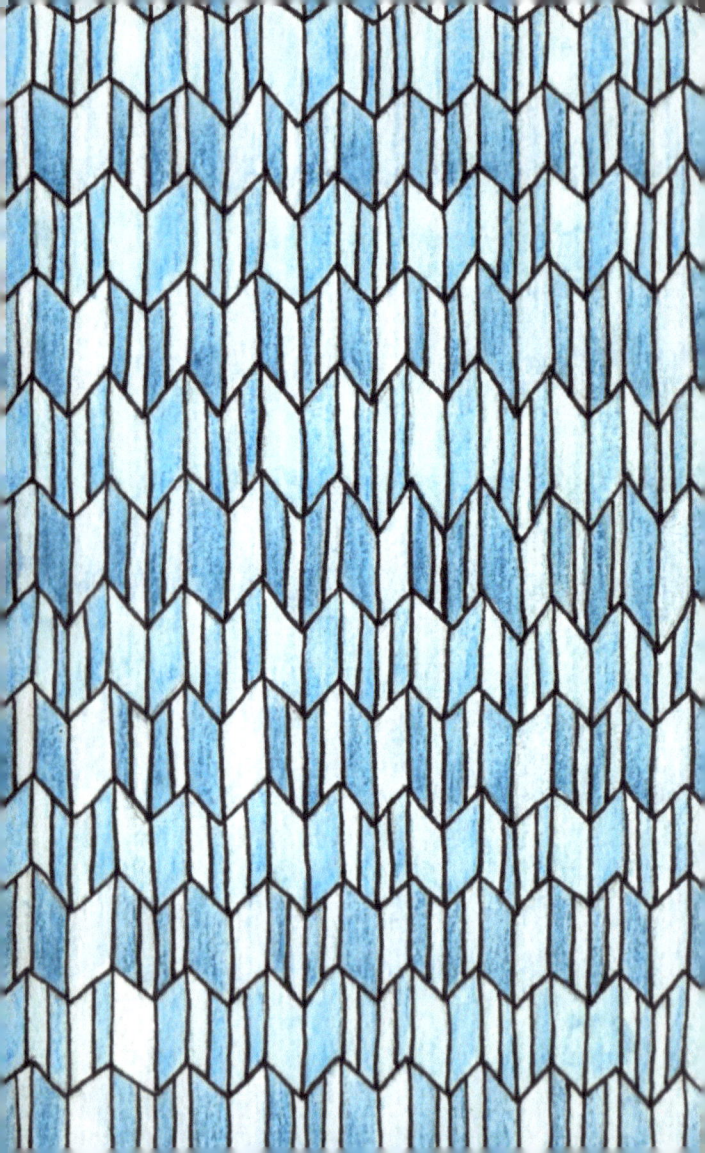

A butterfly passes by …

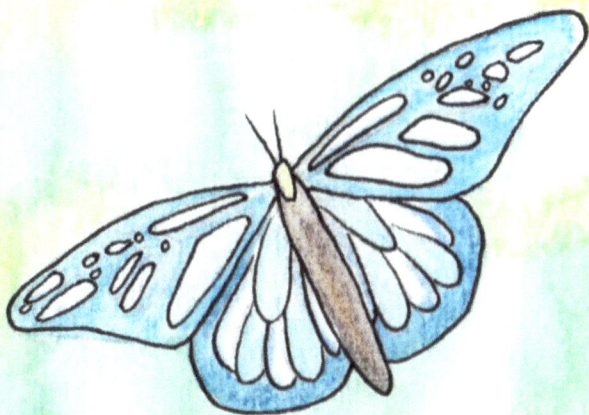

it's blue again

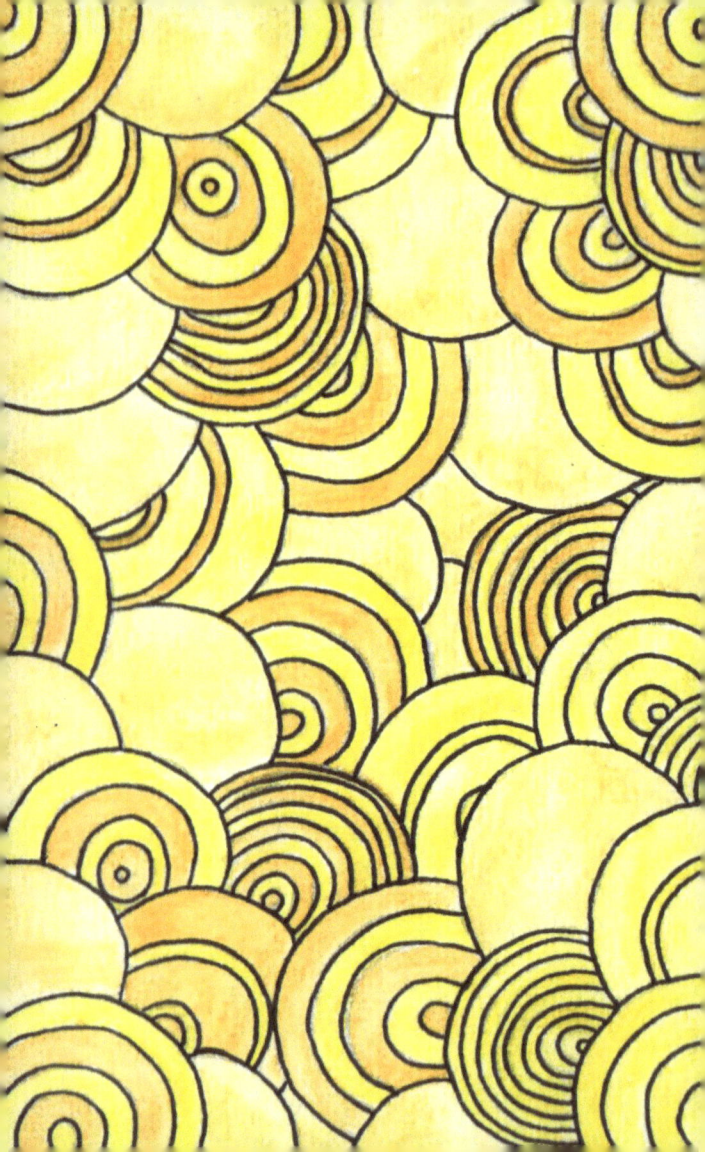

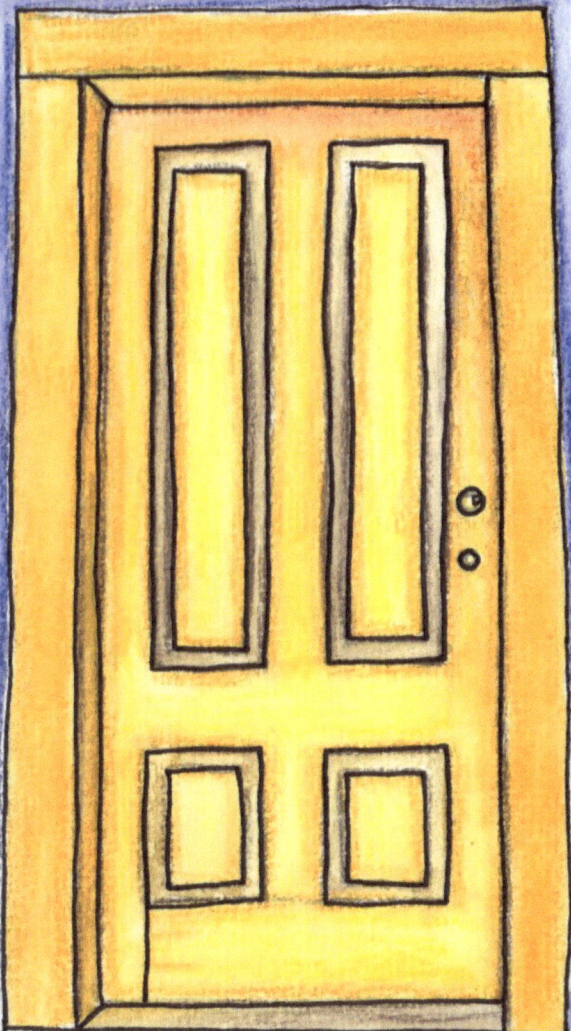

I walk past a bright yellow door

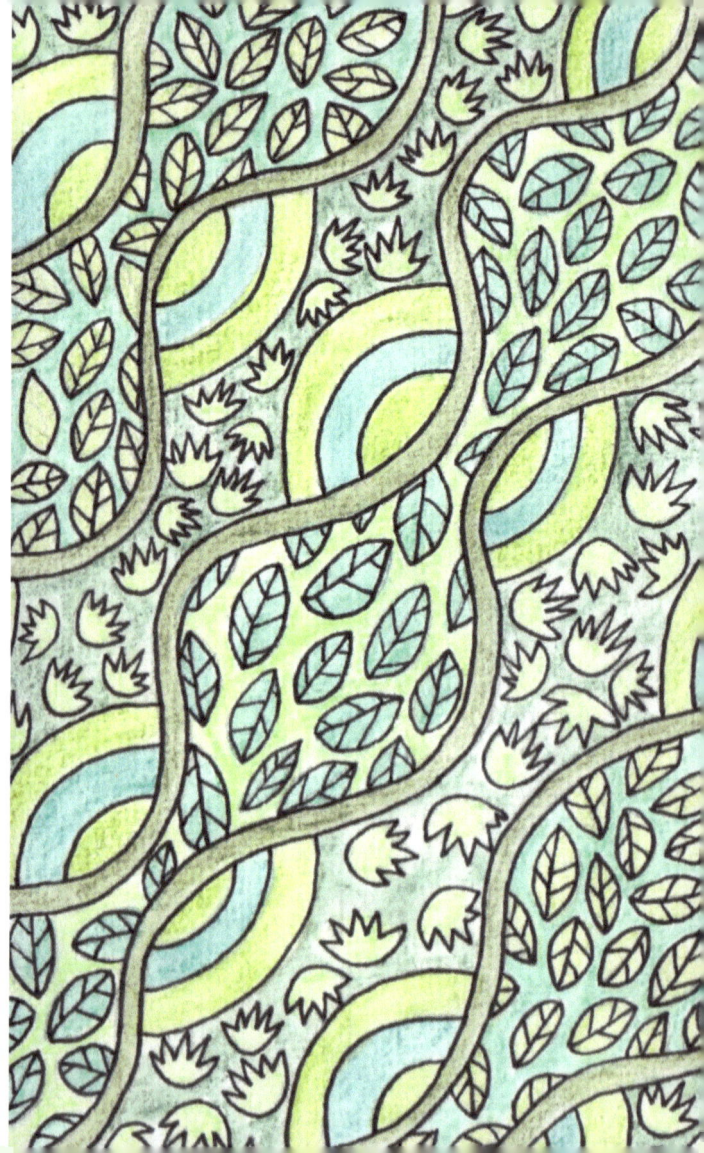

When the sun is red …

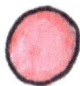

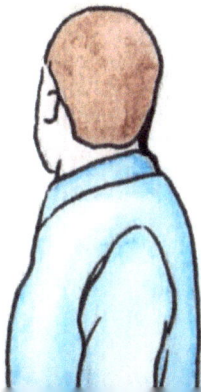

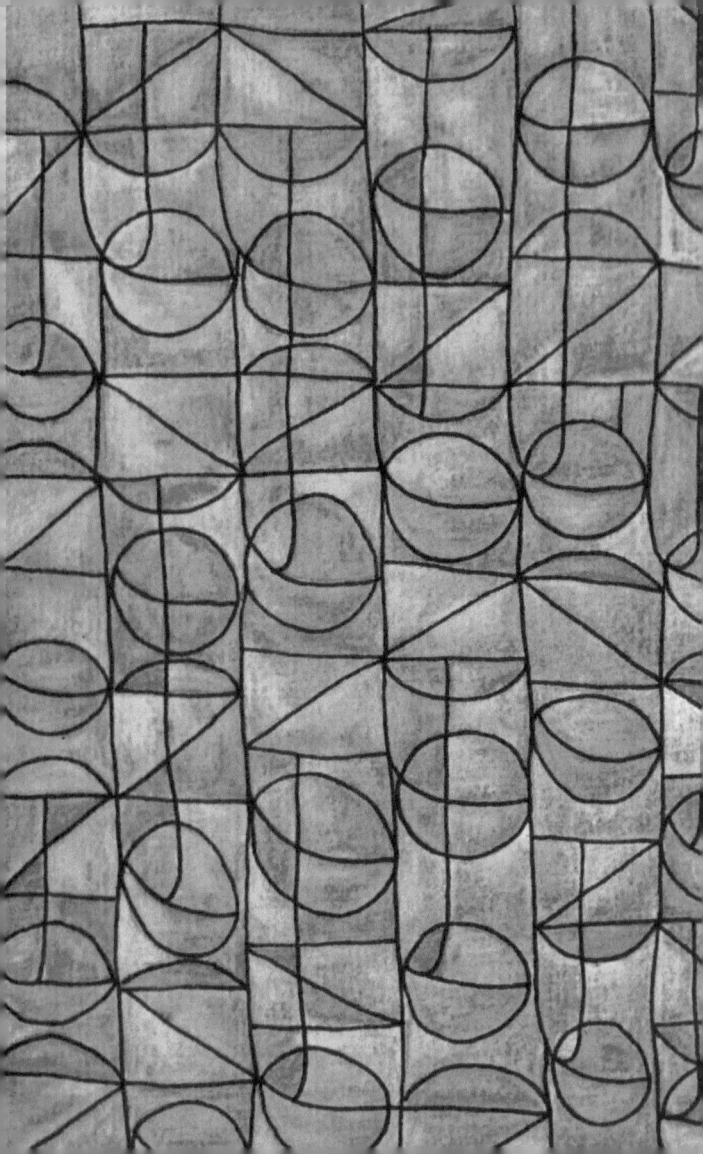

My lunch apple is red

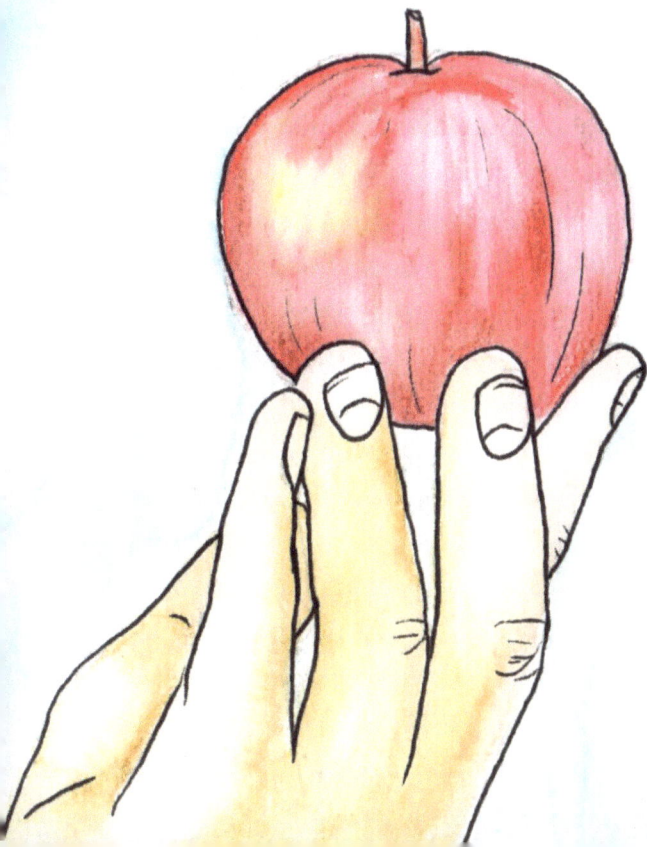

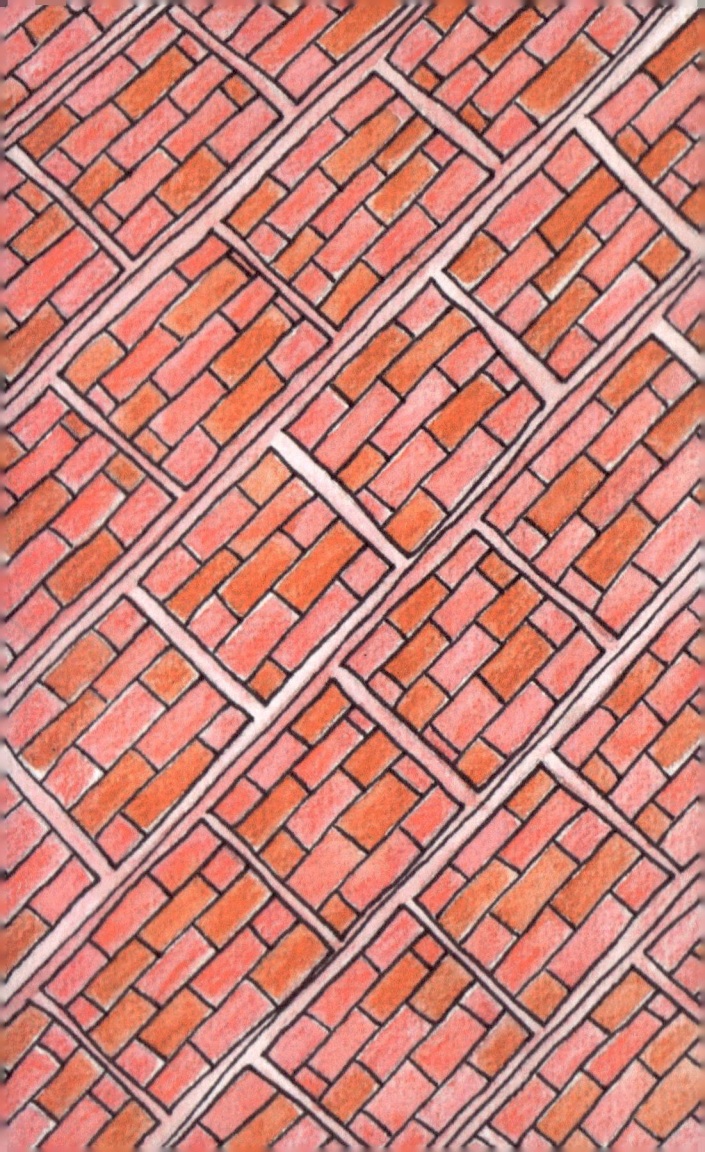

The pencil in my
hand is also red

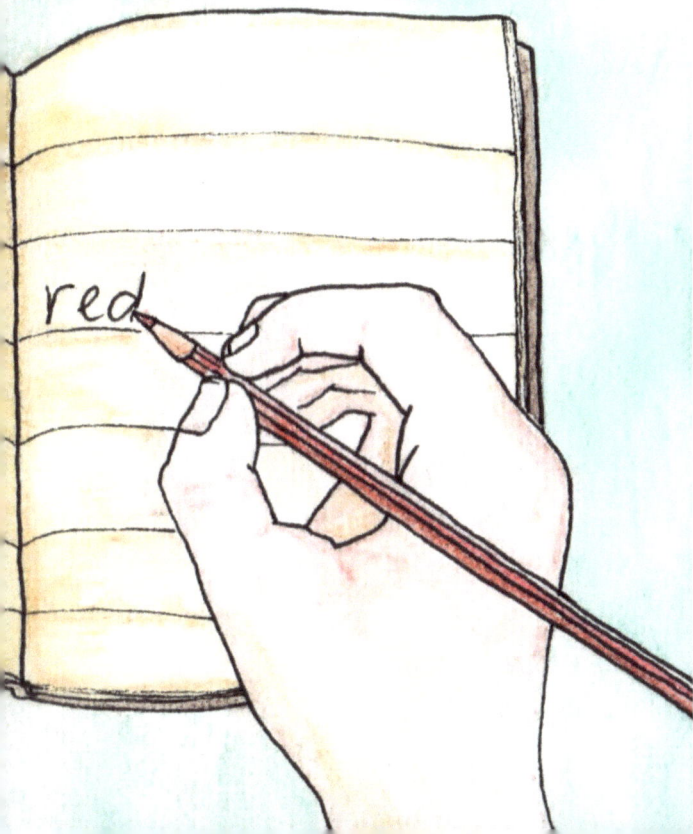

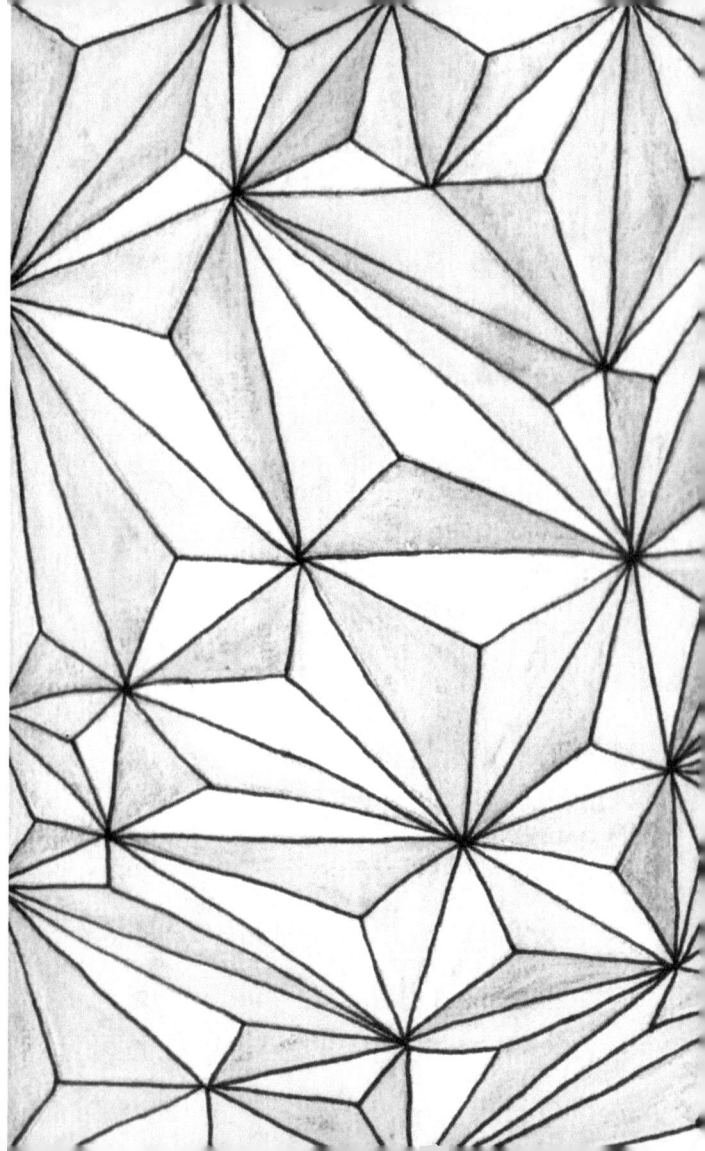

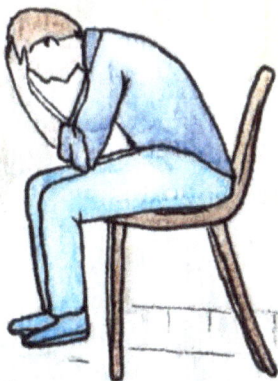

... but I still feel blue today

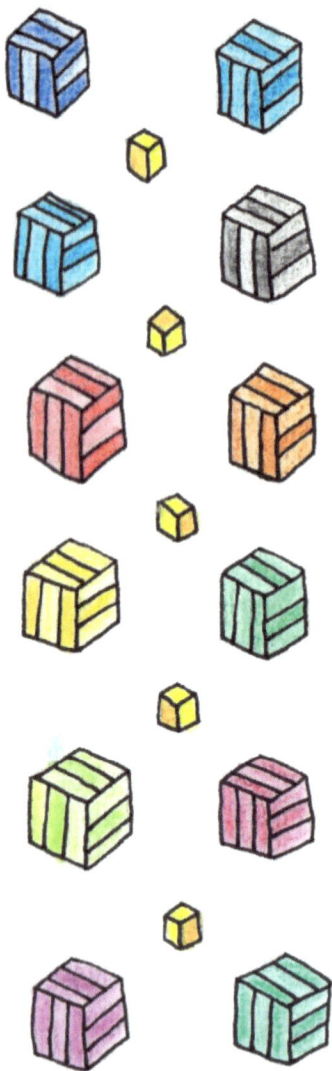

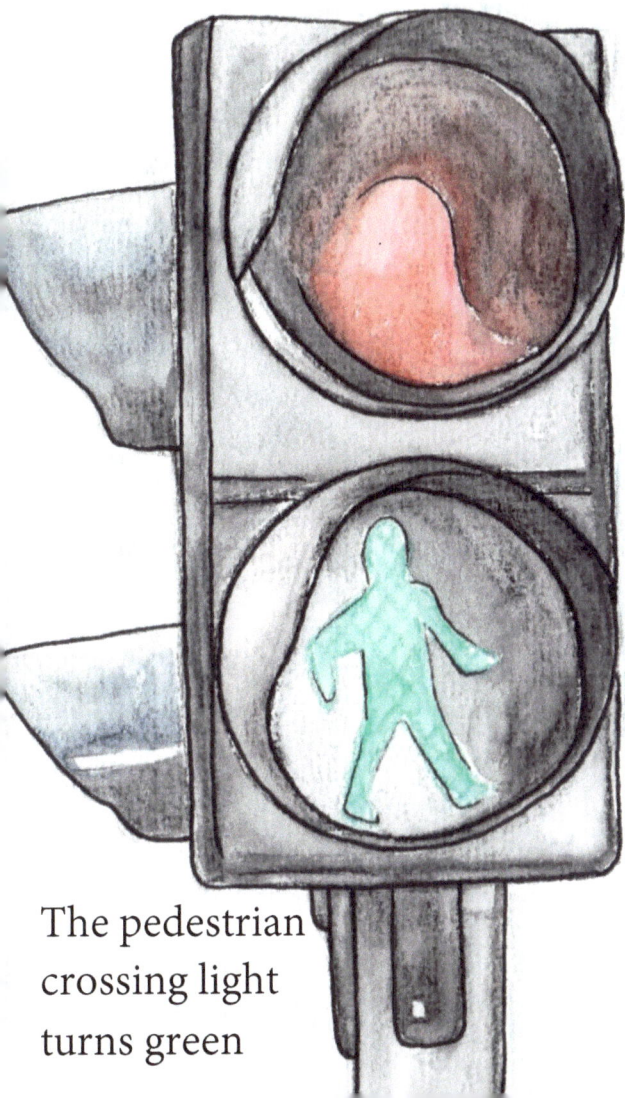

The pedestrian
crossing light
turns green

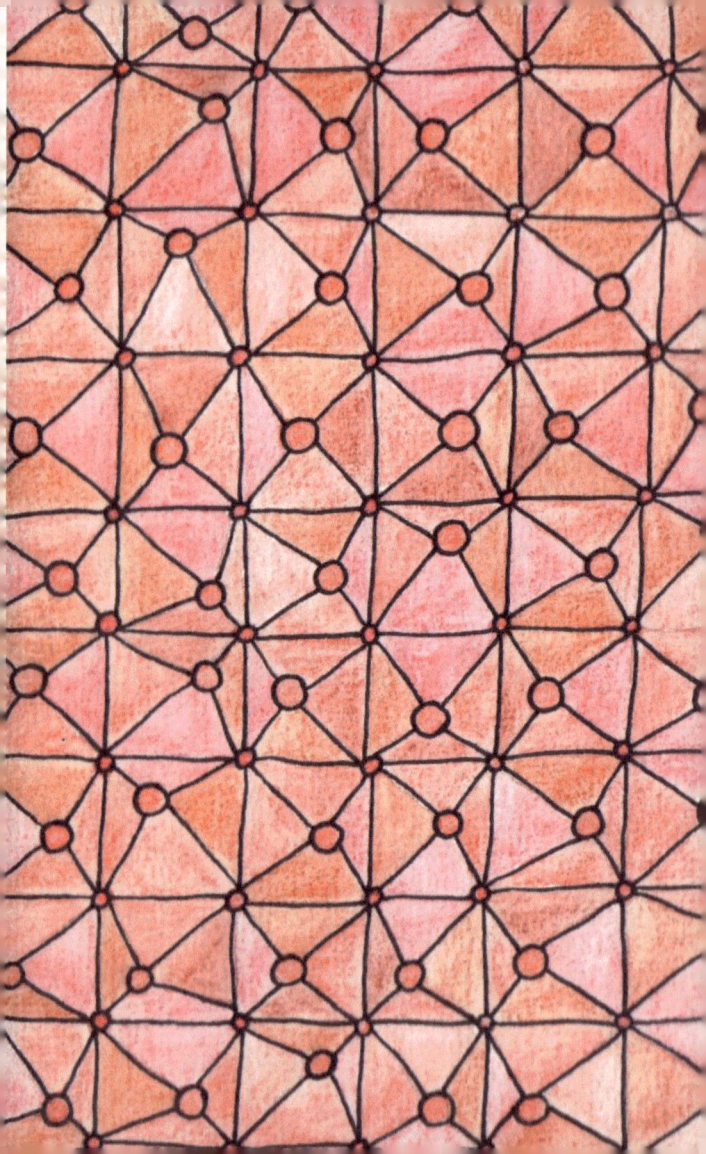

The shoes on my feet are red

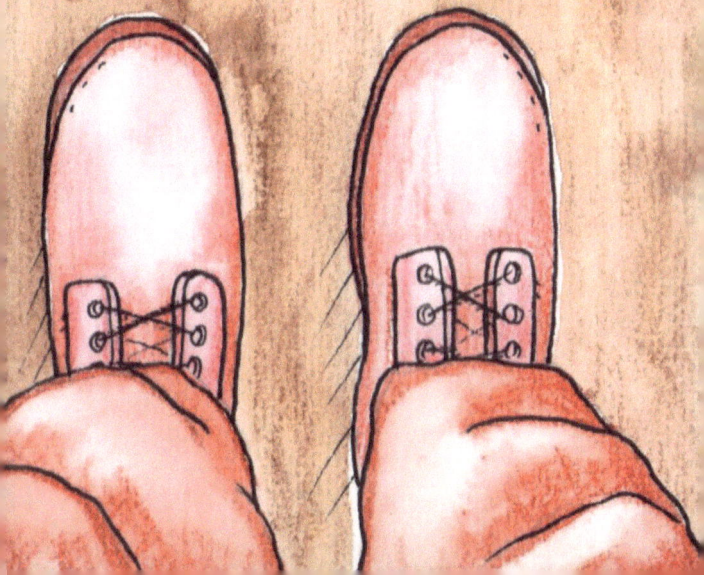

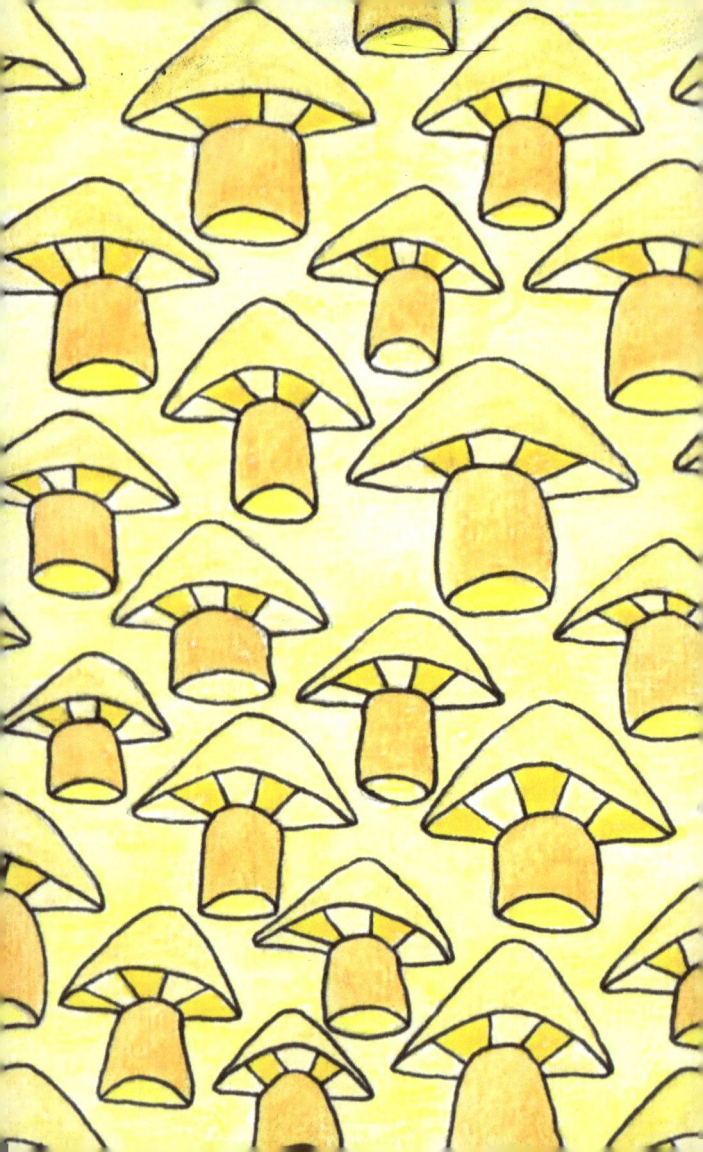

I notice …

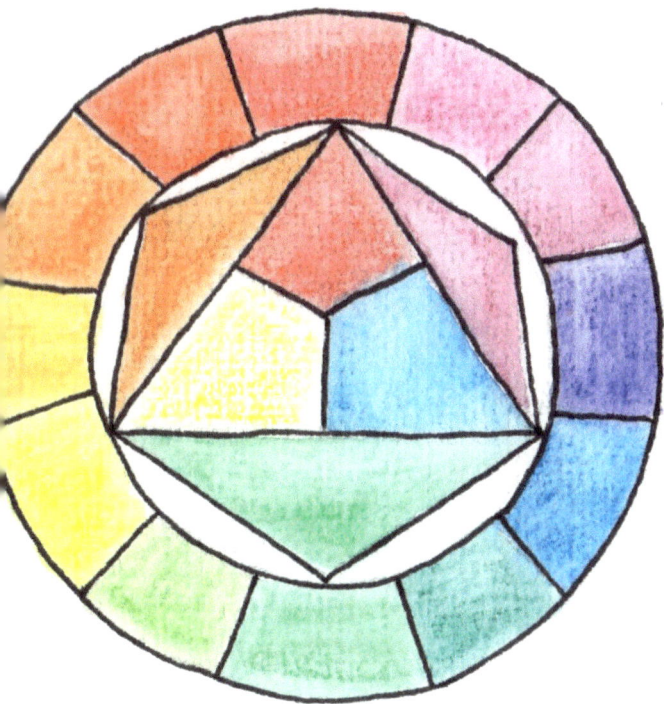

more colours

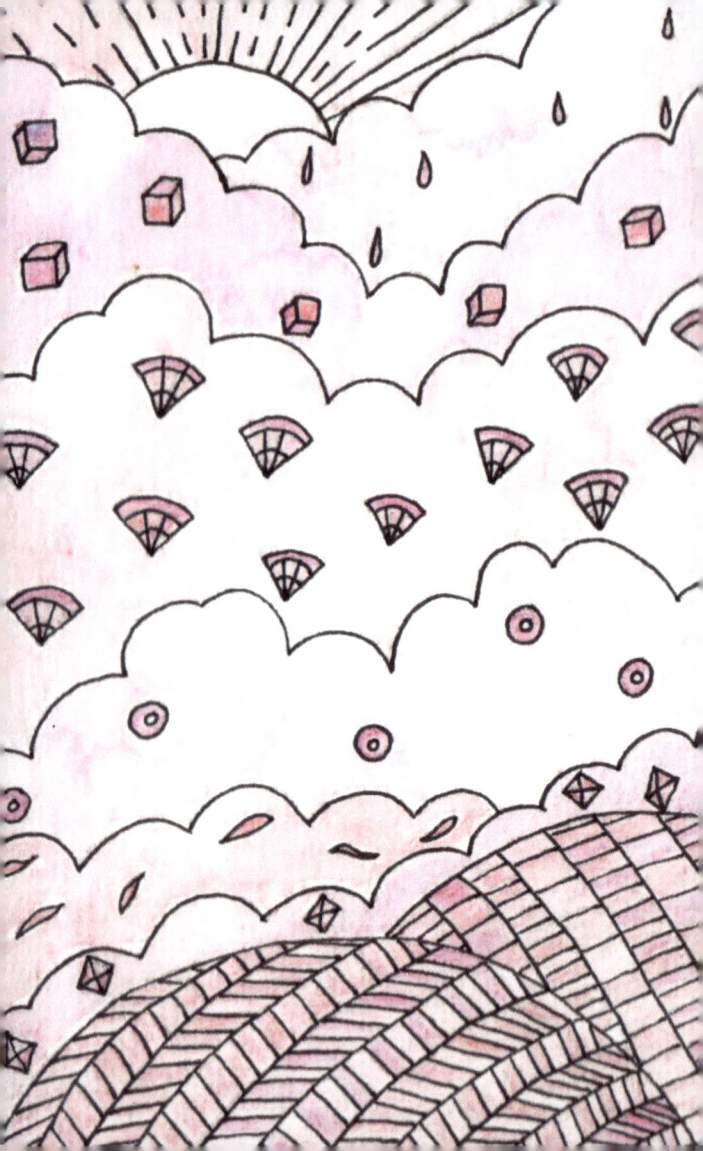

I arrive home
to warm
yellow light
in my house

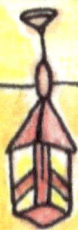

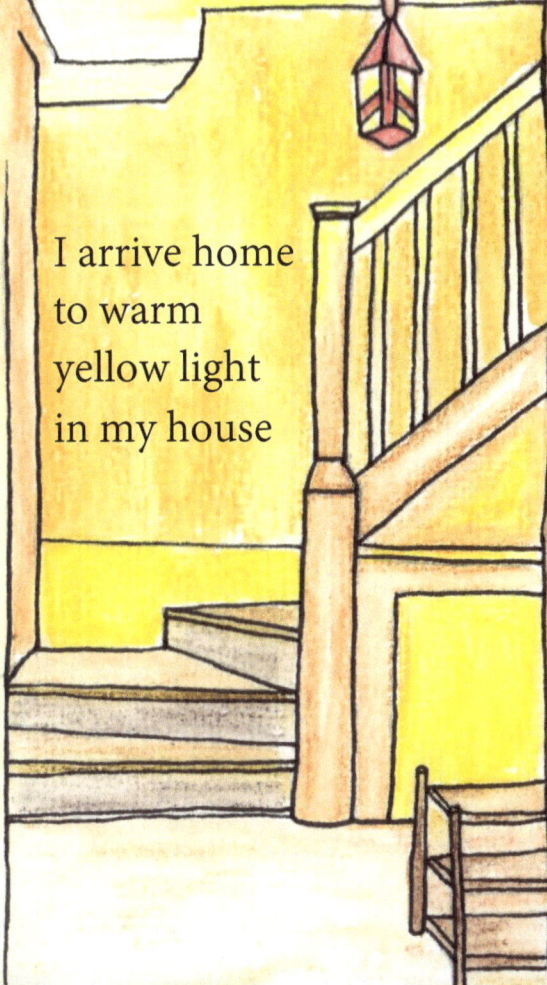

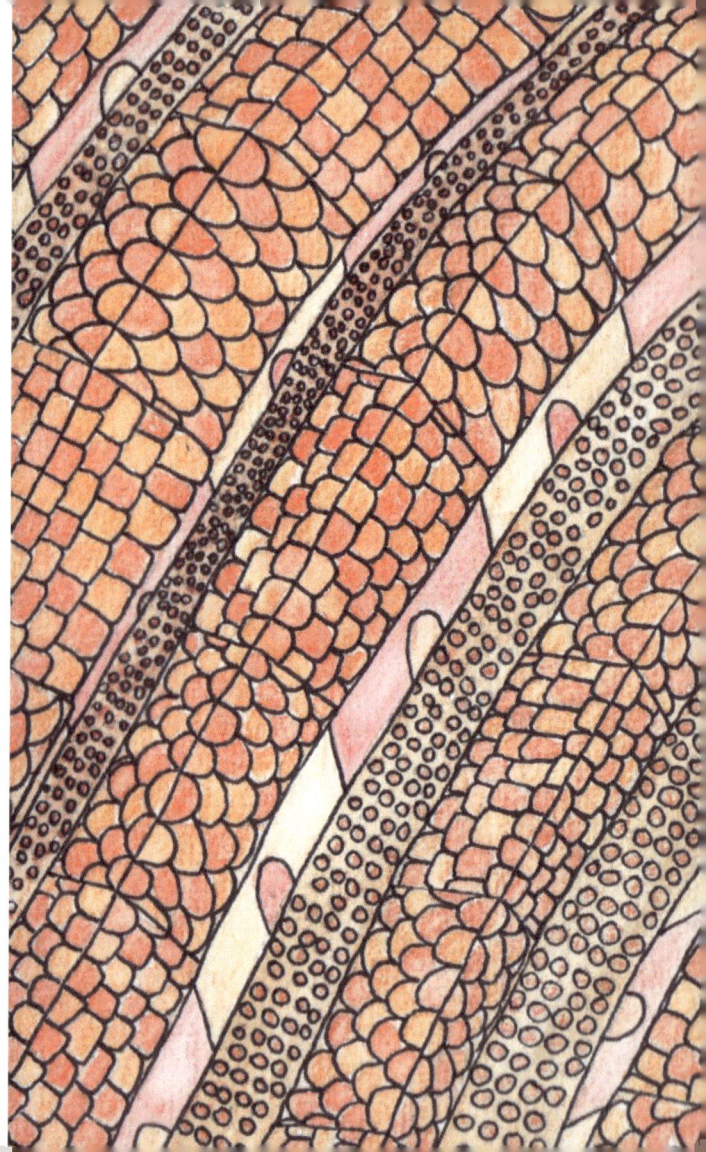

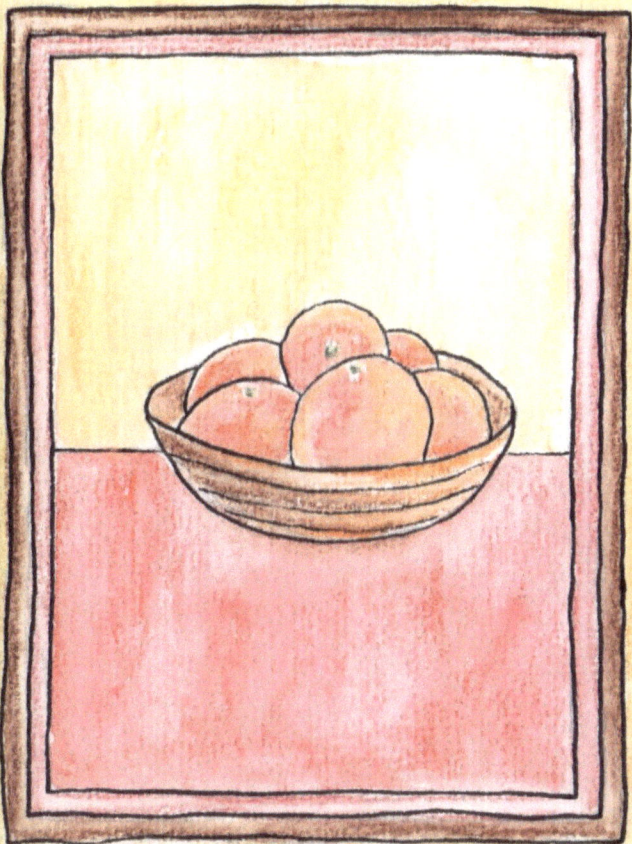

A bright orange painting on the wall

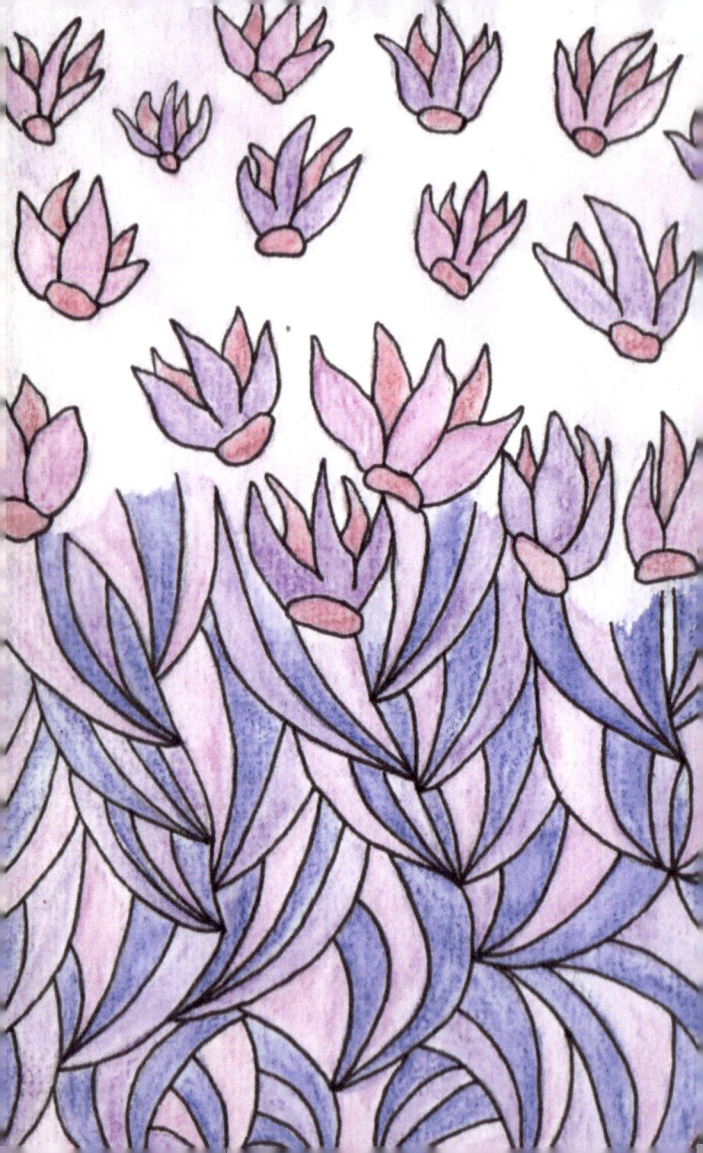

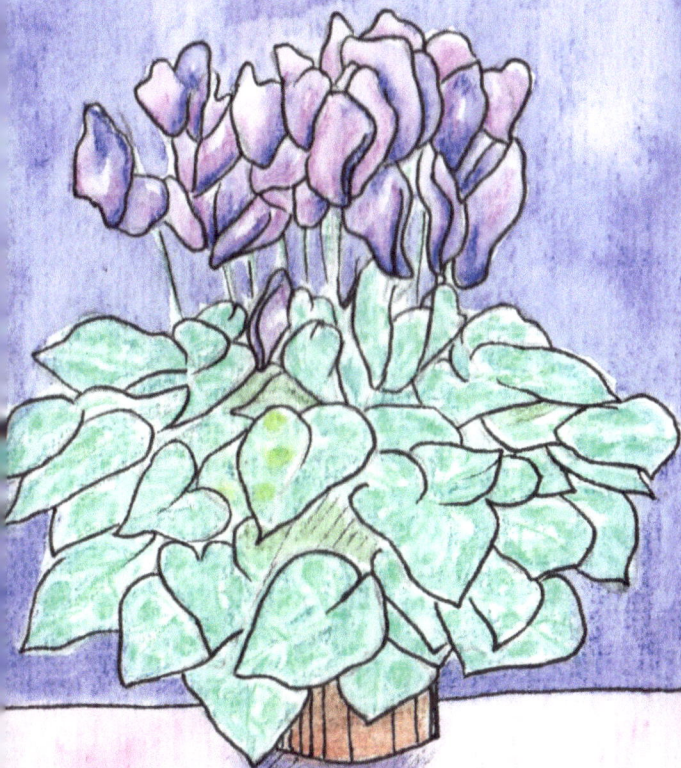

A purple cyclamen in my hallway

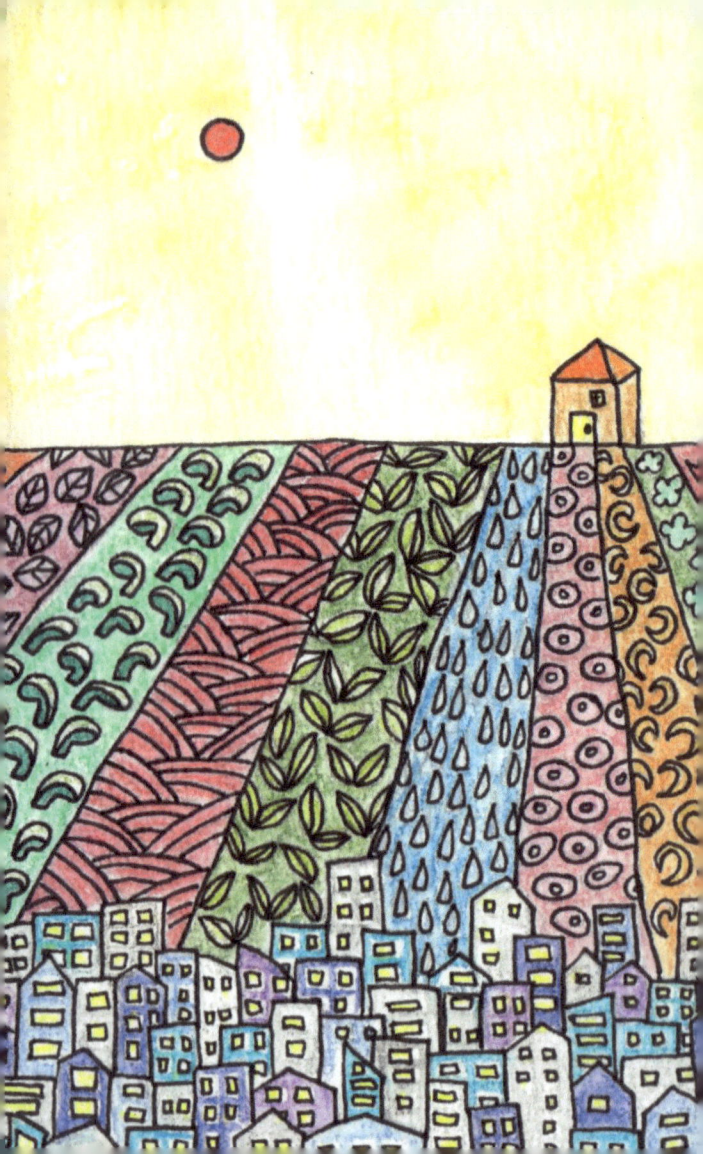

I see my reflection
in the mirror …

I'm not blue
anymore

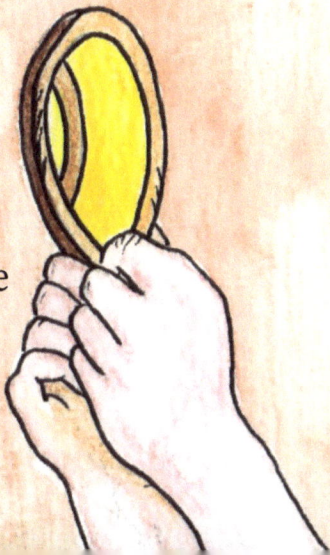

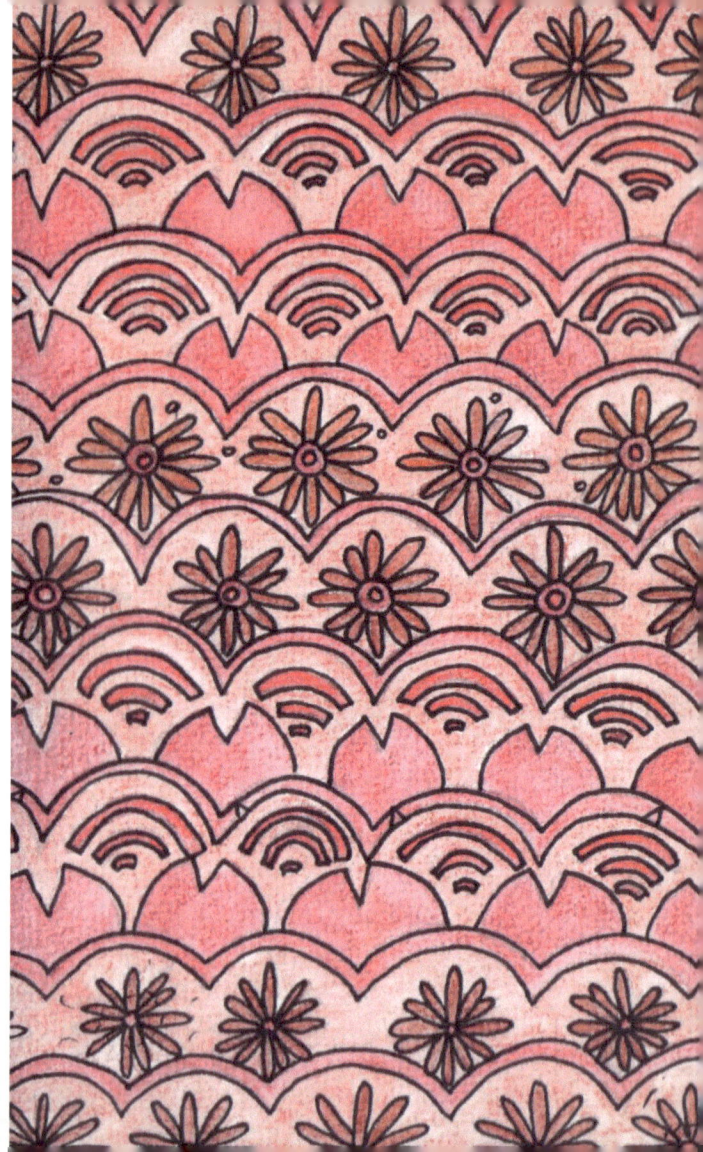

I slide into bed.
Lights are out and it's
black all around.

But now I feel I'm a warm red.

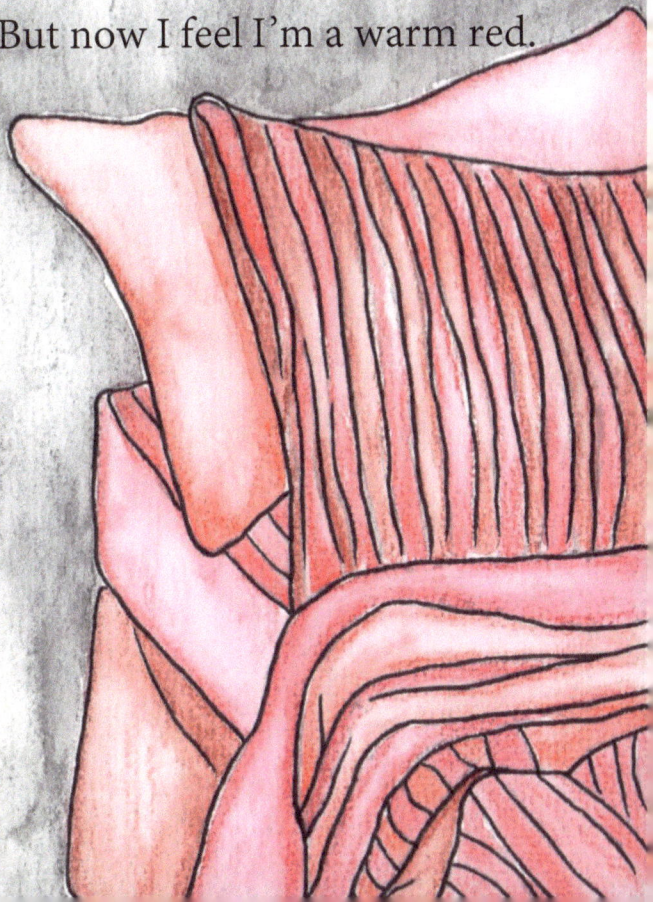

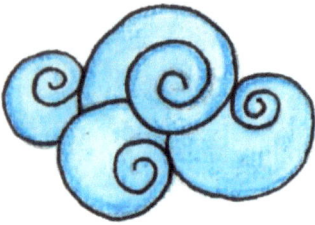

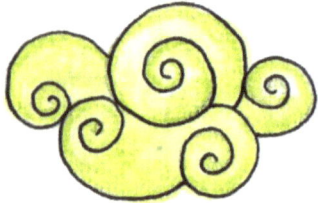

Grey green yellow or blue
whatever the hue that clouds you
that warm red can find you too.

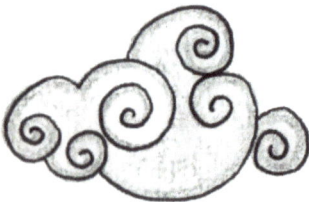

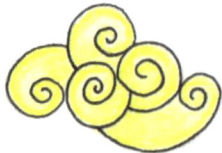

<u>Diary</u>

The colours I found today

Date   Colours

____   _____

____   _____

____   _____

____   _____

____   _____

____   _____

____   _____

____   _____

____   _____

____   _____

____   _____

____   _____

____   _____

www.ingramcontent.com/pod-product-compliance
Lightning Source LLC
Chambersburg PA
CBHW040930030426
42334CB00002B/25